PT 101

ONE HUNDRED AND ONE LESSONS FOR FRESH FACED PERSONAL TRAINERS.

OLI SMALLWOOD

Self-Published by Oliver Smallwood @thepttrainer

This book is inspired by fitness, change and progress and all the epic students I get the pleasure to help start a career.

This book is dedicated to my past, present and future students. Your efforts ignite me, and your ideas inspire me.

CONTENTS № 1

STORY TIME

In May 2017 I set myself the task of writing one piece of advice for personal trainers per day for one-hundred and one days. I'm done, having just printed and read through all 101, and it's 28 October 2019. Late for sure, but eyes still on the finish line.

What's funny is … I'd set the goal, broken it down into small manageable chunks, like we're told to, and, guess what? I didn't do it, and that's OK. When we set goals, we set them with the obstacles, restrictions and parameters that we have at that moment. Things change, people change, and we adjust. So, whilst not writing this book for the last couple of years, I learnt to adjust. I learnt how to deal with the unexpected and I learnt how to stop emotions turning into states. Now, my own personal experience put alongside my journey as a fitness professional, I believe, has led me to have one hundred and one outside the box pieces of advice to share.

WHO IS OLI SMALLWOOD?

I AM A FITNESS educator, teaching the Level 3 Personal Training diploma and a variety of other recognised entry qualifications to students both face-to-face and online.

I'm not a natural academic. I left school with more strings on my Squire Stratocaster than GCSEs, and it had two strings missing. But I do have a tenacious curiosity that gets me by. I like to make fitness education fun, memorable and actionable. So, I've made it my purpose to make fitness education less dull and actually quite amazeballs.

WHY THE BOOK?

HAVING TAUGHT THE Level 3 Personal Training qualification for many years as well as being a personal trainer myself prior, I'm very aware that not everyone makes it. Let's consider the term 'makes it' to mean "turns passion, knowledge and qualification into a career."

I've been fortunate enough to train some fantastic coaches. As with any classroom, I've had students who have just scraped through the course, lacked vision and felt that perhaps their path was already paved for them. Sadly, the majority of these individuals are now either no longer in the industry or they are – but they're moaning about it. I've also had students with vision who also put a lot of effort into the course and are now incredibly successful. There's no real correlation with how well someone does on the course and how well they do as a personal trainer but there is a relationship between how much *effort* is applied on the course and the quality and quantity of their personal training career.

The majority of students I have taught, however, tend to fall into a different category to those mentioned above. This category is made up of talented coaches who have achieved the relevant qualifications and are now in the industry but still need some real support - some advice that's more substantial than "go out on the gym floor and speak to people." It is these people who have led me to write the book. If you are one of these people, this book is for you.

HOW TO USE THIS BOOK?

THIS BOOK CONSISTS of 101 short chapters. Each chapter is a lesson you can apply to yourself as a personal trainer. Some lessons are short sharp tips, some are longer to form strategic advice while some push more of a mindset shift that fresh personal trainers often need. Some may be of instant use to you, some may not be applicable to you, and others you may need to ponder over for a while. Read it all in one go or pick it up 101 individual times; just be sure to add action to the information.

#1

CONDITIONS WILL NEVER BE PERFECT.

THE RIGHT TIME is never going to appear. Waiting for the right moment is like waiting for every traffic light to be on green, all the road works to cease, and the speed limit to be taken off before you leave home. No one has the perfect job waiting for you. No one is going to give you clients. Anything worthwhile is earned.

Consider yourself working the gym floor waiting for the right moment to approach a gym member. Hesitation stands out like a fart in a yoga class. The feeling that prevents us making the decision to pursue something is doubt. Doubt is just an uncertainty towards something – learn to recognise that feeling. The only way to overcome doubt is to act. Through action you will gain certainty, whether that certainty is the outcome you wanted or not. Once an outcome is gained, you can't feel the same doubt anymore, as your question has been answered. The only way forward is action.

One population that will join me in the classroom are people changing careers. I'm often told, "I've wanted to do this for 15 years; I wish I'd done this sooner."

We can learn from these anecdotes. Late is better than never… and no time is better than now.

This pattern of behaviour can be seen in our clients wanting to better themselves but leaving it until Monday. What has Monday got that today hasn't?

#2

GIVE A DAMN BEFORE THEY'RE YOUR CLIENT.

TREAT GYM USERS and followers online as if they're a client already. Care about their goals, their stories and offer advice on overcoming their barriers. Showing that you do give a damn is one of the most likely assets to get someone to buy your service. If someone achieves their goal through your advice and they're not a paying customer, view this as a positive. They will always sing your praises and may be a paying customer in the future.

#3

CONDUCT A CONSULTATION WITHOUT SAYING "LIKE," "Y'KNOW," "AHH," "UMM" OR "ERM."

LIKE, Y'KNOW, ERM ... I mean, it's hard... it's hard to get clients when you, umm, talk like a complete cabbage.

#4

KNOW WHEN TO LEAVE.

I OFTEN TALK TO fresh personal trainers about being at the gym 'full time' when they first start. Whilst I stand by this, you also need to know when to back off. There will be a point each day, or week, when potentially there are no more fish in the pond.

Too much available presence can devalue your service - as the more available you are, the more common you appear. You can also fall prey to the 'sunk cost fallacy'; this is where the more time and emotion you put into a pursuit, the harder it is to abandon it. For example, if you've spent a large amount of time on the gym floor and have not developed any leads, you can be tainted by your emotional investment and may stay to try and salvage something from your time outlay. Have you ever had a friend who has stayed in a relationship because of the amount of time they've been with their partner? Is how long you've been doing something a good reason to continue if it's not working?

Make sure you're giving gym members time to experience their gym sessions without you. Temporary withdrawal can make you more talked about, and potentially more respected. After all, absence makes the heart grow fonder and, as humans, we often fear our losses more than we value our gains.

#5

HAVE A GIGGLE.

Humorous situations are easier to remember than ones that weren't very amusing; this is because humour causes more emotional arousal. The most memorable personal trainers are the ones who you can hear, along with their clients, laughing when you enter the gym. You can bring humour into your teaching points, cracking an egg between your bum cheeks to get those glutes firing, for example. I've seen fun personal trainers establish client bases much faster and with more retention than the most knowledgeable. There is nothing worse than a personal trainer who knows their biomechanics, nutrition, endocrine system, trains well themselves but has the banter of a cress sandwich.

#6

KEEP TABS ON YOUR POSTURE.

I'M SURE YOU'RE aware of the importance of posture in terms of correct alignment, limiting wear and tear on joints and preventing fatigue due to low muscle efficiency. Remember, as personal trainers we are judged by the way we look whether we like it or not - and bad posture looks sloppy.

#7

ONLY ASSOCIATE WITH HAPPY COLLEAGUES.

Avoid associating too much with unhappy, negative or complaining colleagues. Unhappiness is like an infection – don't let it spread to you. This happens particularly when you, as a personal trainer attending to your clients, can allow your mood to be dampened after a negative conversation.

Identify the people you need to avoid and the people you can learn from. Never be rude; just keep them at arm's length. Minimalism expert Joshua Fields Milburn says, "You can't change the people around you, but you can change the people around you."

#8

REPETITION IS THE MOTHER OF ALL SKILLS, AND CONFIDENCE IS THE BY-PRODUCT OF REPETITION.

"Repetition is the mother of all skills" was coined by Tony Robbins. Once you find what works, just repeat it. The repetition will cause the habit to be ingrained in you. This could be something as simple as saying "Hi" to people as they enter the gym. You may have to take it slowly at first, but eventually you'll exude confidence as you welcome them. Confidence is the result of repetition. So, get your reps in with consistency, and eventually you'll be winning.

#9

A DRIVING INSTRUCTOR NEVER DEMONSTRATES A CAR CRASH.

When demonstrating an exercise to a client, keep your sessions efficient by only showing them what you wish to see. In reverse, never demonstrate the wrong technique. You often will see what you show.

This sort of coaching is often seen during planks and press ups with beginners. "I don't want this (hips down) and I don't want this (hips up). I want this (hips parallel to shoulders)." All you, as the personal trainer, need to do is show what you do want (hips parallel). If you don't get what you want, you can correct whatever it is you're shown. Too much information when introducing an exercise to someone, can give them the idea that it's a 'hard' exercise before they've even begun. Keep your explanations at three to five points with beginners, focusing on what you do want to see.

#10
OBSERVE WITH PURPOSE.

LOOK OUTSIDE YOUR locality for market research. If you look to a larger city and notice the trends that are occurring, you'll be able to predict the next 1-5 years of change in your area. This is where social media can be an excellent tool as you can search areas without physically visiting them. Success leaves evidence – find it and utilise it.

#11

HAVE LIFE IN YOUR HANDSHAKE.

A GOOD FIRM HANDSHAKE to seal any partnership is important. There is nothing worse than a limp, lifeless, soggy flap of a handshake. Then again, your handshake shouldn't dominate the receiver - it should suggest equality. Don't spend all day practising, but make sure you have a respectable shake.

#12

COACHES FOR COACHES.

As a coach, don't be afraid to get a coach. Whether this be for your fitness or business development and organisation. Receiving coaching for your own health goals can seem a bit backward. However, it can be a very smart thing to do as it allows you to learn from the other professional's processes.

Getting a coach for developing yourself as a trainer could save you years, although it can come at some expense. To understand some lessons, you do need to experience them yourself. In some personal training positions, you are given a personal training mentor. Whilst this is beneficial, every other personal trainer in the facility will have the same tuition. Rather than use the same standard techniques as your colleagues, look for information from another resource – as you have done by picking up this book.

#13

CONTROL TIME; DON'T LET TIME CONTROL YOU.

ALWAYS BE IN control of time. Don't let your clients see you flustered or impatient with time. Be at every session before they are. Showing you can't keep time shows you don't have control of yourself. Jocko Willink once said, "The only way to get to a place of freedom is through discipline." The more discipline you show in regulating your daily schedule, the more freedom you will acquire.

#14

KNOW YOUR SPIEL.

Ever been asked the question, "What do you do?" and heard yourself give a mumbled, uncertain, flop of an answer. Yeah, me too. Now's the time to sharpen your knife and have an answer as to what you do, what your purpose is and how you create value. So, your task is to be able to summarise your work in one to two sentences.

For example, you may say, "I'm a personal trainer dealing with real world weight loss, aiming to reduce obesity in the UK" or, in my case, "I'm a personal training tutor, aiming to bring the highest quality coaches to gyms in the UK, whilst providing resources for sustainable fitness businesses." Make yours short, sharp and unique to you. There're a lot of personal trainers: what makes you different?

#15

USE VOICE INFLECTION.

Voice inflection refers to changes in the pitch and tone of our voice. We all do this naturally, some more than others. At school you may have had a monotonous teacher who always complained you weren't paying attention. Little did they realise they were partly at fault for not using vocal variety to hold your attention. Now, I liken inflection to when you are highlighting important words or phrases in a book. That's exactly how you should use your voice when coaching. Emphasise the important points to your clients.

#16

THE MORE YOU DISRUPT THE LAND, THE MORE SPECIES WILL LEAVE.

When working the gym floor, be wary of approaching the same individuals again and again. The more you pester members, the more ingrained their no will be. "No" is a complete sentence. Gym users do not owe you any more than that. So, consider your floor-based work the sport of fishing rather than a game of duck, duck, goose. Dangle the most patient, approachable bait you can muster and allow the fish to swim.

#17

SELF CERTIFY.

WHEREVER YOU GO and whatever you do, there are always going to be individuals who have more knowledge and experience than you, and others with less. Often, the 'itty bitty shitty committee' in our own head gives us an internal dialogue that forces us to believe that we're not worthy of an opinion and that we shouldn't share our thoughts. If you really think about it, we need to pass on information; otherwise the information is lost.

I personally find that as soon as I start purposefully educating, via putting on small seminars and teaching qualifications, I start to really understand all I have previously learnt. There is a lot of power in saying out loud what you feel – it suddenly becomes real. So, give yourself permission to have an opinion and the internal consensus to share it. People will agree, and people will disagree. Give yourself permission to be wrong sometimes and allow yourself the bravery to change your own beliefs. Your career and life aren't in print; so you can delete what's unwanted, highlight, bold and use capitals for what's important and, whenever you like, you can hit enter and start a new chapter. Do not wait for permission when you can give it to yourself.

#18

WHAT DO YOU WANT INSTEAD?

Re-direct conversations of what the client does not want to what they do want. You'll often ask someone what they want and straight away they will respond with a long list of all the outcomes they don't wish for. Rather than wade through these, simply ask your client what they want instead. You may find with some individuals you have to do this multiple times within a conversation. We cannot achieve goals by talking about what we don't want.

#19

CHECK THE ECOLOGY.

When setting goals with clients, make sure you check the ecology of them achieving their desired outcome. What effect will their achieving their goal have on the people close to them and the rest of the world? This does sound over the top, but it does make the client feel more important. It also gives them another chance to listen to their voice as they agree to the parameters of their goal. Often a client may shy away from an expressed goal because it may change a household or family dynamic, or potentially upset someone close to them. This is understandable. I've had clients laugh in a moment of empowerment – "Barry's just going to have to deal with the new Margret, isn't he?" It's important to check in, as the goal may be achievable with less life disruption than they imagined.

#20

SHOW YOUR VULNERABILITY.

To BE VULNERABLE is to be exposed physically or emotionally. The way I see vulnerability is to have the possibility of a "yes" when I expose myself, alongside the possibility of a "no". To have the possibility of a win, I must expose myself to the possibility of a loss.

Use your anecdotes and struggles to help clients through their own. Showing that you are not bionic will help clients feel supported. For example, if you're a personal trainer who finds keeping up 'good' eating habits difficult, this may be a strength. However, if you find lifestyle changes easy, it's going to be very hard for most clients to relate to you. Truth, courage and authenticity could be strong selling points that you are not currently displaying. If you are acting, reacting, or even subtracting from yourself, you are never going to be the best version of yourself, let alone the best personal trainer you can be.

#21

IF YOU DON'T KNOW, YOU DON'T KNOW.

IF YOU'RE ASKED a question and you don't know the answer, do not be afraid to say, "I don't know." You might add, "Let me get back to you on that." One of the worst things a personal trainer can do is answer a question with some made-up-on-the-spot waffle. You will get found out, people can Google and have an answer in seconds these days. So, if you don't know, you don't know – but you can find out. No one knows everything.

#22

BE HYGIENIC.

THERE HAVE BEEN two occasions in my career where I wish I had told a personal trainer to brush their teeth or have a shower because I'd heard gym members complaining about it. In honesty, I bottled it both times and didn't mention it to them. I bumped into Aaron a few years later and I'm pretty sure he still hadn't washed; I guess this is me telling him now.

Who oversees telling colleagues that they smell? No one. This is because hygiene is your personal responsibility. You don't need to be spraying yourself before each session like an 18-year-old boy chasing tail in his village's only nightclub. Just don't be offending people before you even open your mouth.

#23

BOND WITH THE BOSSES.

If you are in a role where you have a manager, firstly, good luck to you! When working with managers, be sure to make them feel secure and superior to you. If you wish to make an impression on them, do not flout your talents so much that you conjure up fear and insecurity in them. In your work, make the team above you look more brilliant and you will receive more opportunity for this. In roles where you receive a personal training mentor, be sure to make this person feel valued by you. If they're not feeling valued, it's likely they're feeling threatened. When they're threatened by you, they may favour another personal trainer when they have enquiries. Do not outshine the bosses.

#24

TECHNOLOGY IS A GOOD TOOL BUT A TERRIBLE MASTER.

It was Tim Ferriss who I first heard state, "Technology is a good tool but a terrible master." As personal trainers, we need to be considerate of how much of our practice relies on phone applications and computer software. More importantly, how much are we encouraging others to utilise technology in the pursuit of a healthier lifestyle? We must remember that people managed to live healthy lives prior to the advent of so much technology, so there is no need for it to govern us.

As an example, a lot of us - myself included - are fans of 'My Fitness Pal', the calorie and macronutrient consumption tracking app. Awesome tool. It can make an individual aware of what they're over and under consuming in a visual way that's more difficult to understand without it. Arguably, at the same time, this appliance can very quickly master us. I once had a student who didn't eat lunch because her phone was out of battery. So, for you as a coach, just consider what you're advising and who you're advising. Technology should assist your journey, not drive it. Chuck Palahniuk once said, "The things that you own end up owning you", and no one wants to get owned now, do they?

#25

YOU CAN'T FIRE A CANNON FROM A CANOE.

Ensure your clients can stabilise in a movement before utilising the exercise with power. If a movement can't be done with control and is attempted with power, the movement pattern will break.

CONTENTS № 2

#26
PLANS IN YOUR POCKET.

OFTEN WHEN YOU instruct at a gym where you have shifts, you may be asked to take a class at short notice. Class instructors, like anyone else, are partial to pulling a sicky. So, I suggest you have a playlist and a decent circuit plan ready for when this happens. Having a few class plans up your sleeve can not only stop you looking like a complete novice, it can also make you the club hero when Mr Motivator has a last-minute change of plan. Do not fear, if the Zumba instructor doesn't turn up, you don't have to give the people Zumba. Give the members your strengths - unless you're badass at Zumba. Covering classes, last minute or not, is a huge opportunity to make yourself remembered, gain clients and spend the extra cash on heroin for a rainy day… Aha, just checking that you were paying attention.

#27

NEVER GIVE A WHOLE SESSION FOR FREE.

You're in the supermarket, an employee is offering small samples of free cake in order to entice you to buy a whole one. If they were to give away whole cakes for free, no one would buy any. If you give your whole product or service away for free, it doesn't get sold. So, keep your taster sessions shorter in length than your paid sessions, to leave potential clients wanting more.

#28

TAKE PRIDE IN YOUR ENVIRONMENT.

Pride refers to getting pleasure from your own achievements, possessions, an associate's achievement, a personal character trait or a skill you have. Let's consider the gym you work in your possession. It doesn't matter whether you own the gym or just work there; treat the gym with it's equipment as if it's your possession. You are responsible for it, so take pride in it.

When you are tidying the gym, you become very apparent to the members. This makes it known that you're not training anyone at that moment, and so you'll find more members will approach you. If gym users are of the correct mindset, by seeing you make the gym a well-functioning tidy environment, they will help maintain it too. It's easier to get clients when they see you're proud of the environment that you're training them in.

#29

ONLINE IS THE SAME AS OFFLINE.

When we're on the gym floor, we can't expect to walk up to a member, offer them personal training and expect them to say yes within 30 seconds. We must begin with meaningful engagement. More likely, a few meaningful engagements spread across multiple occasions. I've had clients sign up who've been considering having personal training for six months to a year. Let's get one thing straight: clientele is never instantaneous.

Online is the same. You cannot expect to put out one post offering an 8-week program and for someone to sign up within minutes, without any value given beforehand. Again, you've got to meaningfully engage. Gary Vaynerchuk, a social media expert, refers to this process as "jab, jab, right hook." This is where we provide lots of jabs, which can be described as content that aims to engage and trigger an emotional response. Following a selection of jabs, you come in with the right hook, which is where we sell or promote ourselves. So, even when you're selling your services online, you need to meaningfully engage.

#30

MEMBERS ARE ALWAYS WATCHING.

Just before you head off to the office to sit down and flick through your phone. Just before you sneak off to the toilet, not needing it, merely escaping the public eye. Just before you pop to get a coffee at the café, despite just finishing one and possibly not even needing another. Just before you publicly tell your colleague how bored you are. Just before you complain about your management, or the payment structure you signed for. Realise this... Members are always watching, often considering personal training, and guess what? They aren't going to consider a fidgety, complaining, bored clock-watcher dressed as a personal trainer, who they haven't seen assist anyone in months of their working there.

#31

STOP SAYING YOU'RE OVERQUALIFIED.

Personal training is not a career in which you can become overqualified. There is one basic qualification you need to do the job, your Level 3 Personal Training Diploma. Anything you do from that point on is another badge that simply enhances your practice.

I've often heard trainers brag about their degree, or the strength and conditioning qualification they're taking. Whilst I'm all for studying in higher education, it doesn't over-qualify you. Degrees, workshops, certificates and online courses may, however, help you develop a specialist area. Still, they're not over-qualifying you. The question I pose is, at what point does someone become overqualified at helping someone else?

#32
VISIOBIBLIOPHOBIA.

Look in all directions. There is no-one you can't learn from, even if the lesson is 'what not to do.' It's easy as a trainer to fixate on the actions of trainers with a lot of experience, a large online following, or all of the qualifications. We can gain from looking at more established trainers, BUT it's not the only direction to look.

Are you a trainer who's fearful to post on social media, but wants a voice? Are you concerned about being 'called out' by the 'experts' for getting something 'wrong'?

Well, you're focusing on the wrong population!

The direction to look in is the people that you wish to serve. What do they need help with? What seems misunderstood? Are they doing dumb ass stuff that's ruining their progress, which you could change in a minute's video?

You are sharing something that you know, with people that don't know and people that need reminding. Your position is important; what you know is important; you are important. We could ponder all day on the pros and cons of social media, or we could use it as a tool to our advantage: helping others.

#33

FIRST NAME TERMS.

> "A person's name is to him or her the sweetest and most important sound in any language."
>
> ~ Dale Carnegie

ADDRESS CLIENTS AND potential clients by their name, not 'Mate', 'Buddy' or 'Pal.' Being on first name terms promotes respect in a relationship. This is especially important in the meetings you have with individuals prior to them becoming a client, showing that you remember – and care.

This is just as important in text or email. Lead with the first name; it shows that this communication was meant for them. We're personal trainers, so let's be personal.

#34

RESPECT OTHER TRAINERS' SPECIALITIES.

SUCCESSFUL BUSINESS IN fitness is all about relationships with the right people. For me, I didn't have any experience in competing in triathlons or long-distance running, so I had a colleague that I'd refer people to for endurance event training. In return, he would send over a lot of the real-world weight-loss clients that I enjoyed working with.

It takes time to build these relationships. At first, it's hard to turn away clientele but, for sustained happiness at work, concentrating on goals you're interested in is essential.

At first, it can be a balance between focusing on 'what you want to be known for' and putting food on the table. If you're not the right person for the particular solution, you may gain more business from passing the client on. Build these relationships, respect other trainers' specialities, and they will respect yours.

#35

ATTEND A REGULAR NETWORKING GROUP.

If you attend a regular local networking group, you'll find that you can pitch yourself in that group as the go-to personal trainer. Often, networking groups only allow 1-2 of each profession, so the ratios can be on your side. You'll find you meet people from all industries, which will allow the floodgates to open for you. Networking is another way to create meaningful engagements, and as sales and leadership expert Tim Sanders says, "Your network is your net worth."

#36
STAY AUTHENTIC.

We all want to be happy, right? To be happy, there needs to be alignment between our thoughts, discussions and actions. A sure-fire way to NOT be happy is to be inauthentic: to copy, to steal and to lie. Ok, there are going to be similarities in the ways that we and others in the industry do things. There are going to be fixed principles that a lot of personal trainers share.

Just make sure that you're delivering your message your way. Avoid copying other personal trainers' marketing material, videos and social media content. You're not aiming to be a shit cover band and you are not going to be able to do someone else better than they can.

#37

BASIC BITCH BIOS.

You've always been into exercise and been playing sport from a young age, haven't you? You've spent three years studying sport and exercise, haven't you? At weekends you like to get outdoors, read a book and spend time with friends? You're all about lifestyle balance, aren't you?

Of course, I'm being facetious. There's the harsh reality that the outline of our journey to becoming a personal trainer may not differ that much from another's. So, be sure to focus your bio on what does make you different and what does make you the right person for your target audience.

The client is reading your bio not your memoirs, so keep it short. Write it in the first person, in the way you'd speak in real life; this helps the client get an idea of how you communicate. Utilise the words that the general public would use; your bio doesn't need to include references to "DOMS" or "EPOC."

Make sure your bio has a call to action. If this is online, it can be a click through or book in. If this is on the wall at your facility, make sure it invites the person to approach you.

Make it fun and honest. Robin Roberts, the American television anchor said, "Your mess is your message." So, make it messy and get people curious.

#38

THE GOOD, THE BAD, OR THE DIFFERENT.

Avoid labelling things good or bad. This teaches clients there is a wrong and a right when really, they are just different. For example, are gummy bears bad? Well, it depends what we're aiming for. If we want a fast hit of sugars, gummy bears could be useful. If we're looking to be nourished, perhaps there are options better suited. Not good, not bad, just different.

You'll often find there's a relationship between a person labelling good or bad and their lack of knowledge and experience on that topic. You'll also find a connection between a person who labels other people good or bad and their level of insecurity.

#39

INFORMATION BOOKLETS.

Having a relevant well-presented source of information to pass on can be priceless. You're having a conversation with a member in the gym and you can say, "Pass me your email; I've got a booklet on this that you may find interesting." How many personal trainers have written short booklets that they're actively utilising as an engagement tool? I'd say less than 10%.

You can also use a booklet online to attract members to join your email list. Instant free quality help that, once created, doesn't cost you any more time.

The time it takes for you to write it will be completely worth the business and reputation you receive for your efforts.

#40

HOST AN EVENT.

From a weekly nutrition seminar to an annual fitness day for a local charity, events are important. They will boost your following and get you known for the right reasons. I used to do a weekly nutrition seminar and would regularly gain clients from it.

Thinking big and creating a local 5k run or a more varied fitness challenge could be massive in terms of your learning curve and building clientele. Regardless of what it is you choose to do, if it shows the public that you're willing to stand up-front and present your knowledge, or create opportunities for yourself, it's a good idea. Visibility is the modern-day credibility.

#41

RIGGED.

Now, it's a touchy subject but we must address the rig.

If you're positioning yourself as a fat loss trainer, try to not be obese. If you're positioning yourself as a strength coach, it helps if you're strong.

Knowledge, qualifications and confidence are all powerful things. But, whether you like it or not, this is a very visual industry and the majority of your prospects are going to allocate some of their judgement to the way you look. Aubrey Marcus, a podcaster, author and business owner says, "To be of service, you must be fit for service."

In a period of growth, I asked a client why he'd chosen to train with me. He said, "Your body looks obtainable." My first thought was, "You prick!" I asked another client – similar answer. It turned out that part of my success was because my body looked like other people could achieve it. A lot of my clientele became exactly that – men who wanted to look slightly better than average.

The real question needs to be, "Would you pay for training by you?" If you're answering no, it could be due to the way you look. You haven't got a problem – you've got an opportunity.

#42

MEDIAL ARM FOLDS AND RESTING BITCH FACE.

WHETHER YOU'RE IN a session or working the gym floor, stop folding your arms. It displays boredom; it's a barrier to communication; it shows that you're not conscious of your surroundings. "But it's comfortable!" So is wearing a onesie and eating ice cream whilst watching The Lion King, but guess what? That doesn't get or keep clients, either.

Make sure the intent your body language expresses is open, approachable and welcoming. Arms by your side, smiling with an upright posture. Try to find the confidence to not have anything in front of you, no desk, no leaning on equipment. If you're available, be available.

#43
MIRRORING.

BUILDING RAPPORT IS a vital skill for a personal trainer. Being able to form strong connections quickly is a difference that can make the difference.

Mirroring is when we SUBTLY imitate a person's behaviour. This could be a physical thing (e.g the position someone is sitting in), a vocal thing (e.g. the rate at which someone is speaking) or a language thing (e.g. the type of words a person chooses to use). We can adapt ourselves to show them we are responding positively.

This can happen subconsciously. Next time you're on a course, look at how some people are naturally in rapport with each other, sitting in the same position with their feet tapping at the same speed. This often means people are subconsciously agreeing with each other.

So, we know that when body language is the same between two individuals, a positive connection has been formed. Therefore, what we can do is copy what a person is doing to grow connection.

There are three ways that we can mirror. Mirroring itself: this is when you copy a person as if you are a mirror; for example, if they move their right arm, you move your left. Matching: this is where you do the exact same as they; if they lift their left leg, you lift your left leg. If their volume gets louder, your volume gets louder. We can also cross match, which is a less obvious method. Cross matching is when you make a corresponding, but different movement to mimic someone's actions. For example, every time they scratch their chin, you tap your finger. You'll be able to tell if this has worked if you tap your finger and they respond to the tap by scratching their chin.

When you're in consultation, take these skills on board. The client is sat back in the chair, you sit back in the chair. The client smiles, you smile. Have a play with this. My advice would be to try it out in low risk situations first, such as family and friends, and see how it goes before taking it into your practice.

#44

SELF-DEPRECATION.

I once had a student who was bright, new to exercise, young as well as driven, willing to ask questions and very curious. She had an excellent sense of humour, often making me LMAO when I was supposed to be teaching. When it came to her practical exams, she'd introduce an exercise and then criticise her own technique. Whilst self-deprecation can be amusing, in your case when you're deprecating the service that people are paying for or considering paying for, this could be dangerous territory. If you were going to purchase a phone and the salesperson said, "It's not the best phone but I'll show it to you anyway," you're unlikely to buy that phone.

Embrace the stage you're at on your learning curve, be excited that there's so much you can learn. It's a cliché, I know, but sometimes you do have to fake it to become it. Avoid introducing an exercise saying, "I'm not the best at this…". Demo using the regressed version of an exercise until you're confident about using a standard version.

#45

CONTEXT OVER CONTENT.

Observe the context more than the content of a situation. By context, we're referring to the circumstances and facts that surround a situation and, by content, we're referring to the substance of a speech or information being made available. The context will always hold more importance than the content, as context defines content.

You may see a personal trainer using a certain exercise – that's our content. You may think, "Why on earth is your client doing that?" But you don't have any circumstantial information, the context, to have an informed opinion. This is one reason I'd advise you to be wary of judging another trainer's choice of exercises for their client. You only know the content and not the context of the choice - and it's probably going to be of more value to focus on your own stuff anyway.

#46

THE 3 E'S: ENTERTAIN, EDUCATE AND EMPOWER.

As a coach you need a good balance of the 3 E's.

Entertain: can you tell a gripping story that's funny and relevant, or an analogy that's going to make your client spit their protein shake out?

Educate: can you teach without being 'the teacher', making people feel comfortable on your level, so that they look forward to learning more from you?

Empower: can you take the entertaining, educational anecdotes that you're providing and get the client to turn it all into action?

One thing I've learnt from tutoring in the classroom is, learning is much easier when you're laughing. Doing is much easier when you're focused on doing, rather than being done. A lot of trainers focus on increasing their knowledge, which is epic, but not many focus on how they communicate that knowledge. So, can you entertain, educate and empower?

#47
TREND STACK.

TREND STACKING IS when you add two or more successfully selling things together to package a more unique product or service. The biggest trend stack of the last 20 years is coffee and wi-fi. What's the fitness equivalent? We can often use trend stacking when searching for specific populations, for example, 'strength training for climbers' or 'yoga for powerlifters'. Build a good solid stack to build a good solid client base.

#48

DON'T DEVALUE YOURSELF.

Discounting demonstrates a lack of confidence in your service. It says my service isn't worth what I usually say it is; it's worth less. When you're discounting as a personal trainer, you are discounting you. You're saying, my knowledge isn't what I originally said it was, my banter is worse and I don't put in as much time behind the scenes as I should. Cheap is not good and good is not cheap.

To attract clients without degrading yourself, create comparison within your packages, which makes one option seem like good value when sat next to others. For example, you may say, "I'm £90 for one session, but I offer 10 sessions for £500." Services are not to be discounted; products, however, can be. Personal training, of course, is a service.

#49

SELL WHAT THE CLIENT WILL INSTANTLY RECEIVE.

WHILST IT'S GOOD to sell the long-term benefits of your services, when you're trying to get a potential client across the line focus on the immediate gains. Through signing up to you, they are instantly gaining structure to their training, for which they don't have to make any decisions. This is huge. People can get very stressed and confused by not knowing what step one towards their goal is. When someone signs up to you, ask yourself what immediately changes for them? Sell that!

#50
CLEVER INCENTIVES.

Offer good, interesting, valuable incentives that don't diminish your worth. As an example, rather than offering 12 sessions for the price of 10, offer the 10th session as a bring-a-friend session. This Is fun; it makes the client want to get fit to show the friend how far they've come. Also, at the end of the session another person knows about your services, and they're probably going to tell more people about you. After all, word of mouth is still king.

CONTENTS № 3

#51

MAKE MEMBERSHIP YOUR MOST ATTRACTIVE PACKAGE.

THE MEMBERSHIP MODEL of business has become increasingly popular within the last few years. If we're constantly selling session packages, like a 12-week plan, for example, we need to consider the life span of our customer. Sure, some people may buy package after package but this won't bulletproof your bank balance. We can create a better set up for both client and trainer by encouraging direct debits – let's call them memberships; sounds sexier.

This is less financially invasive on the client, due to making smaller payments more often. It also creates a routine of paying and receiving, so the client naturally factors the cost into their general outgoings. We should never expect a client to be a client forever but a lot of goals take time. For you, the trainer, you can put in a clause of one month's cancellation notice as a minimum, making it much easier for you to look ahead with security.

#52

DON'T SELL PERSONAL TRAINING.

IF PEOPLE ACHIEVED the goals they desired, they wouldn't invest in a coach. It's important to note that very few people buy personal training because they want a personal trainer. People buy personal training because they want an outcome, like losing weight, getting stronger or gaining accountability and training structure, for example. Sell these outcomes to your potential clients rather than selling personal training.

#53

DON'T COUNT YOUR CHICKENS BEFORE THEY'RE HATCHED.

Only believe what you know to be true. If an individual books in for a consultation with you, that's an individual booking in for a consultation. If someone buys a personal training package from you, that's someone buying a personal training package from you. A consultation may lead to someone investing in personal training, or it may not. Often, we self-talk, sometimes even telling others about all the clients that are just about to sign up. From training personal trainers, I've notice most of us assume we will gain more clients than we do. So, don't go changing plans based on outcomes that haven't materialised yet.

#54

CONTENT MARKET.

Create and share online material such as videos, blogs, and social media posts that do not explicitly promote your brand but stimulate interest in your products or services. For example, if you're a trainer and you talk about the benefits of having a trainer or share the workout you did that day, you're not directly marketing your product, but the content is likely to lead people to your services. It's less of a shove, more of an arm around the shoulder – "I'm here if you need me."

#55

YOU CAN'T REPLACE THE BASE.

Outside of the base of your normal clientele people may come and go, but your base or your "tribe" as some personal trainers call them, will stick by you. When you're established and thinking about adding more clients, first consider if there's something else you can offer your base.

Consider how a football team has fans with a club shirt who may visit once every 2 years. What about season ticket holders? What about the fans with a season ticket who get their hands on every piece of merchandise that their club produces, and travel the world to see every game? Find the same enthusiasm in your clients, and produce for them. Ask them what they want more of, whether that be guides, videos or more classes and seminars. There may be more profit in the base than adding more clients, as there is no cost to promote to the former. 20% of your clients could result in 80% of your income.

Whilst we're considering Pareto's 80/20 law, we should consider the problematic 20%. This is the portion of our clients who cause most of our headache - cancelling last minute, never being quite happy, complaining of expense, not washing their gym kit. Sack them, recommend another personal trainer to train with them and save your energy for your base.

#56

UTILISE THE DECOY EFFECT.

I FIRST DISCOVERED THE decoy effect in Dan Ariely's book *Predictably Irrational.* This is when customers change their preference when given an additional option that alters the focus of what's the best value.

Let's take popcorn, for example. If we had two options, a small at £3 and a large at £6, most people would get the small because they'd view the large as too expensive.

Now if we add in a medium, our decoy, at £5.50 then most people will get the large because it appears to be better value. Who's going to buy a medium when you could have a large for only 50 pence more?

So how do you apply this to your personal training biz?

Imagine you currently offer 6 sessions for £240 (£40 per session) and 20 sessions for £750 (£37.50 per session). Most people either aren't going to purchase either or will buy the £240 package, as £750 is a large payment in one instalment for most people. Selling the smaller package is not ideal, as you'll end up having to ask for money more often.

We can add in a mid-runner, for example 12 sessions at £450 (£37.50 per session). By doing this, the

20 session package has become a decoy - it's the same price per session as the medium but more payment in one go. It therefore makes the 12-session package seem more appealing and will lure prospects to purchase this package over the others.

You can utilise this principle with any product or service you sell, whether a package or a membership. You could even take two friends out on the town with you, one that looks nothing like you, and one that looks like you (but not as good looking) thus giving prospects something to compare you to. Having the ability to compare can cause a bias towards something we perceive as more attractive. You will find this tool very useful in your pricing structure.

#57
WHAT, WHY....

TELL THEM **WHAT** they need to do, tell them **why** it will work, *sell* them **how** it's done.

Ever been searching through the internet for information and something just seems to be missing? It's probably the how. For example, you will find lots of YouTube videos on calorie deficits, what they are and why they work. BUT, to find out how to create a caloric deficit will require some form of commitment, whether that's an email address or wonga. This is important. If you're not using **how** for financial gain, use it to gain a communication line outside of social media, the easiest being an email address.

How is where the power is. **How** is your product or service. **What** and **why** are your infotainment to get enough of people's trust and respect to consider committing to your **how**.

#58

EXERCISE YOUR NECK MUSCLES.

Nod your head whilst speaking and whoever you're speaking to will be more inclined to agree with you. This nodding has also been proven to make you feel more confident in what you're pitching.

Utilise this during your sales process to get a person across the line. With all these subtle non-verbal communication skills, it's important they stay subtle. No need to be nodding like Churchill the dog.

#59
OLI25 (AFFILIATION CODES).

Be cautious about forming affiliates.

To affiliate is to connect or associate with a person or organisation. In our industry this usually involves a commission code. Where you'll advertise a company's product, offer out a 'discount' code to your following, letting the retailer know the sale came from you. You will then receive whatever amount of money was agreed per sale. On paper this can seem like a good extra earner. However, you need a large following to really harness the benefits of these schemes. Regardless of following size, this will likely be a short-term gain. Short term gains can come with long term consequences – ask any Tinder user.

It's tempting to write "just don't affiliate" and that is probably the answer in most cases. However, it's not true of all. If this is something you're considering, make sure you put your values first, and that whatever you're affiliating with is a 'good' product.

One question you may need to answer is whether your values and the affiliating company's values align? Are they honest, or are they preying on the uninformed to make a quick buck? Sadly, this can be true in a lot of circumstances. Like everything, you need to figure the risk-to-reward ratio. You may not get away with selling crap twice.

#60

BUILD YOUR GYM COMMUNITY.

Introduce your clients to one another, to the staff and other club members. This will help create positive accountable relationships that support their goals. Feeling popular in the gym will keep them coming as well as starting a good word-of mouth-referral scheme for you. This can be achieved by offering a circuits class to your personal training clients or having a clients' evening out.

#61

QUANTIFY YOUR CLIENTS' PROGRESS.

Make sure that you're tracking your clients' progress regardless of whether it's a body fat reading, 1RM squat or plank time. Often, these small progressions can't be seen by the beholder, so make them visible with numbers.

#62

SPEND TIME ON THE BUSINESS AS WELL AS IN THE BUSINESS.

Don't spend all of your time personal training. Make sure you have a section of time each week that you devote to improving your business. In large offices they often have a breakaway area to discuss new ideas. Create this area for yourself and go there, at least once a week, and make things happen.

#63

COLLABORATION IS INNOVATION.

Looking for clients is one part of the equation; looking for relationships is the other. Look for relationships that benefit both parties. The kind of people to look out for are:

- People that you can learn from.
- People with a customer base.
- People with products that could be useful to your clients.
- People that you're going to enjoy working with.

A collaboration doesn't always have to be with another fitness professional. There may be a local café that you can team up with, who knows? When you collaborate with another business you bring two sets of customers together - and often they multiply.

A good way to figure out the organisation or personnel to co-lab with is to ask yourself the question, "Who has my clients?" As an example, female personal trainers in the city I live in will deliver HIIT classes in the local high-end women's gym-wear store. Even if they're doing this for free, this is a good decision as it's putting them in front of potential clients who are willing to pay £100 for a pair of leggings. So, they're unlikely to be fazed by personal training prices. Collaboration is innovation.

#64

BE YOUR OWN LABORATORY.

Make sure you're taking your body and mind through a positive progressive journey. The more you do this, the easier it is to relate to your clients at different stages of their journey. You don't need to be a cover model, competitive athlete or have an ass the size of a house; just demonstrate it with actions that inspire.

#65

SAVE 10% OF YOUR INCOME.

SAVE 10% OF your income to put toward your further education. This doesn't just mean qualifications; utilise it for anything that improves you and your business. It's important you focus on this as a percentage of what you're earning rather than a fixed amount of money. The habit of saving is as beneficial as the money itself, regardless of income. Once you've mastered 10%, consider upping your savings to 20% of your income. Whilst money isn't everything, having some spare change in the bank can help you make decisions without getting stressed about finance.

#66
IT DEPENDS.

A LOT OF ANSWERS to fitness and nutrition questions are "It depends". Be proud to say this rather than rattling off the current BS fads going around. The message really is to be honest with your clients. Tell them what you feel will work best for them given their current circumstance. If it depends, then it depends.

Clients, like anyone else, can suffer from authority bias. This is where someone of authority has shared information and, because they're high profile, we're more inclined to believe it. It's up to us to filter this information to give our clients what they need. We also tend to believe something based on the amount of people that agree. Five hundred people can say something stupid and it's still stupid. Everything is circumstantial and needs context; therefore, it will always depend.

#67
MEMORY MATTERS.

REMEMBERING INFORMATION ABOUT people shows you care. How annoying is it when you're asked your name for the third time by the same person? When a client tells you something in a session, be sure to either jot it down or pop it in your phone notes. David Allen, an expert at getting things done, describes the brain as a processing centre, not a storage centre. The easier something seems to be remembered, often the easier it is forgotten or slightly confused.

For example, your client tells you they're going on holiday to Menorca. In 40 minutes, you're not sure if they said Majorca or Menorca. So, when they get back in 2 weeks time, you're not going to have a clue where they went. Even worse, you ask them why they missed their session last week. Jot it down so you get it correct. Ever forgot your anniversary date and experienced the fury of your partner? If you'd just put the date in your phone, things would have been so different! Remembering shows you care, and we have the tools to assist our memory these days - use them.

#68

TEACH CLIENTS HOW THEY TRAIN, NOT HOW YOU TRAIN.

Your client, most likely, is a different weight to you, a different height to you and probably has a different goal to you. Make sure you're training clients to be the best they can be rather than a subpar version of you. For example, your 80-year-old new to exercise client doesn't need to be shown a low bar, wide stance back squat.

#69

KNOW YOUR AUDIENCE.

THERE'S INFORMATION YOU share with your mates that you don't share with your Mum. There're things you say to your colleagues that you shouldn't say to your clients. Remain professional, whilst being you.

It's important to recognise the stage of development your clients are at. Are you giving them assignments they're ready for? As an example, I once made the mistake of advising a client on a rough daily protein guideline prior to informing them of the foods considered quality protein sources. This client's understanding of protein was powder from a tub. At our next session together, the client told me the difficulty they'd had consuming so many shakes and the amount of time he'd spent, well… in the loo. The penny dropped, and I went back to teach him some fundamentals. Mistakes are for learning from.

Whether it's implementing a lifestyle change or dropping an F-bomb, do the research and recognise when your client is ready, and what information they need to know next.

#70
SURPRISE!

Surprise your clients with communication when they would least expect it. No, not a random weight check in. Send them an article or video relevant to something you had been talking about. This shows them that you are thinking of them outside the sessions. Not many trainers do this; many are stubborn with their time. This also taps into the law of reciprocity. This is where someone does something nice for you, and you have the urge to return the gesture, often to a larger extent than the original gesture… think of the presents.

#71

BRING YOUR COMMUNITY ONLINE.

Consider creating an online group page, for example a Facebook group, and invite clients into it. This will bring old and new clients together and allow them to offer support to one another. This also offers you a fast place to communicate with all your clients as one. You could use this for simple things like your availability and more community building tasks like clients' success posts. We have a lot of tools at our disposal these days; take advantage of the good ones.

#72

BE KNOWN FOR YOUR PROFESSION NOT FOR YOUR CHOICE OF EQUIPMENT.

A KEY FITNESS PROFESSIONAL will understand it's more advantageous to be known for their profession, as opposed to being known for a piece of equipment they favour or class they deliver. Avoid being labelled a spinast or a HIIT trainer. I've even met 'the cable guy' and a trainer that had her clients doing step ups on a vibrating plate – the equipment burned more energy than her clients. Both have left the industry. I'm not saying don't instruct spin classes or utilise HIIT protocols. I'm saying focus on client outcomes.

We have a lot of choice of how to get a client from A to B. Become known for getting them from A to B, not how you got them there. For top-quality trainers, this will differ from client to client. Be known for the journey you took, not the car that got you there.

#73

KEEP YOUR PAWS CLEAN.

NEVER BE THE talk of the town for the wrong reason, or a reason that would be counterproductive to your trade. Look to keep your paws clean. What you do outside of work is your business and it stays outside work. Do not accept physical payments from your clients.

#74

EMPATHY >.

To be empathic is to be able to understand and share the feelings of others. Empathy can create openness. Brené Brown, an emotions researcher, says “Empathy fuels connection and sympathy drives dis-connection.” Unconsciously, sympathy is used to stop someone’s feelings, usually because the person confronted by them doesn’t want to deal with them. This is similar to pity, “Oh, you poor thing!” and consoling, “You did the best you could, and it wasn’t your fault.” Not to forget clichés like, “Cheer up”, “You’ll be fine” and “There’s always next time”, all rather dismissive. They just basically say, “Stop feeling – I can’t deal with your emotions!”

To have and own empathy in your coaching is to understand that what you say probably isn’t going to make the difference, no matter how clever it sounds in your head. It’s to understand that connection will. To be empathic is to be without judgement, to recognise the emotions in others and communicate that, whilst seeing the world from another person’s viewpoint. It’s believed that to connect with others you need to be able to connect with yourself. My cousin is a doctor and he said, during a period when my grandad was in hospital, “I treat every patient like my granddad.” It’s exactly what you should do, i.e. make every client's story dear to your heart. When we really care, our actions will always be right.

#75
IMPLEMENT YOUR FINDINGS.

Reading, studying qualifications, going to seminars and attending networking events are all important. However, none are as important as the moments after. Whilst listening to your current audiobook, jot down the take-home points. Take a note pad to seminars and write down the things that you think can help you improve. In the days, weeks, months and years after all of these experiences, make sure you've utilised the information given to you.

You could do it now with this book. Is there anything you've read so far that you feel could improve your personal training practice? Highlight it, write it down and implement it.

CONTENTS № 4

#76

STOP MAKING YOUR CLIENTS EAT SHIT.

QUALITY FEEDBACK OCCURS when a coach improves a client without telling them that anything was wrong. Focus on what you want, not what you don't want. The shit sandwich (good, negative, good) is the start of quality feedback. However, we don't need the negative point. Try this with your clients:

1. Tell the client something they did well.
2. Tell the client something you want more of.
3. Offer overall feedback.

This may sound like: "Really excellent effort levels today. I'd like to see a little more depth and control on your squats and lunges. Overall, I'm impressed with your progress and can't believe how much your deadlift has improved." By telling the client we want more of something, it suggests they can already do what you're asking, and no one eats shit anymore.

#77

STOP ONE-UPPING YOUR CLIENTS.

"THAT'S NOTHING. WAIT until you hear what I did last weekend!" Shut up and listen to your client.

One-upping is when a person talks about their achievement, another person in the conversation announces how they have already done that, or how they have done something else far superior - and how they were blindfolded riding an ostrich.

Celebrate your client's achievements. Unsolicited comparisons of accomplishment will not retain clients.

#78

COMMON DOESN'T MEAN NORMAL.

THE WORD 'COMMON' means something is happening often. The word 'normal' can mean to conform to a standard. In biology, normal can mean to be free of disease and from a psychological standpoint it would mean the patient is sane. We seem to have got these words completely confused to the point where people are accepting such low standards, because these standards are often seen.

Amongst your client base don't let the common be normal. For example, high blood pressure is commonly seen, but this doesn't mean we should accept it as normal. The same can be said for a postural abnormality – it's common, but it's not the norm.

#79

BE CAUTIOUS OF EXTENDING THE LINE.

You're a personal trainer, remember that. It's very easy to get carried away and decide you're a clothing brand/yoga guru/model/supplement store. Focus on you, the personal trainer. When you try to extend your name elsewhere, it can often tarnish it. The clarity of what you are becomes questionable, and clients may think your interest is elsewhere. Have other aspirations, but those aspirations don't need to fall under the umbrella of your personal training business. If it isn't the same, put it under a different name.

#80
GROW IN KNOWLEDGE, NOT IN IGNORANCE.

> "As our island of knowledge grows, so does the shore of our ignorance."
>
> ~ J.A Wheeler

As you gain knowledge, remember where you started and the obstacles that you had to overcome. It's common for a coach to become fixated on a certain methodology but be ignorant of the fundamentals, or oblivious to a simple comment the client made in consultation.

Little bits of knowledge are great; just be sure not to be insensitive to the client's likes and dislikes. Allow your knowledge to grow, whilst maintaining awareness of yourself and of your client.

#81

IF YOU'VE GOT ONE ASS, YOU CAN'T RIDE TWO DONKEYS.

Clients will often come to consultation with 2 or 3 goals. Your job is to narrow those goals to one until accomplished. What is the focus to be for the next training block? Avoid promising marathon success whilst putting on muscle, or large increases in strength whilst losing body fat. Not because it isn't possible, but because no one can ride two donkeys as well as they can ride one.

#82

INFORMATION OVERLOAD.

CONSIDER HOW MANY people you're following online. If you choose one person's method, be it for business or for nutrition and exercise, stick to it and unless it's a heap of crap you'll be ok. An issue with the plethora of voices available on social media is often due to following one person's plan and adding in bits from multiple influences. You'll end up with a cocktail, and in my experience, cocktails deliver inadequate decisions.

#83

EVERYONE BEHAVES IN THE BEST WAY THEY CAN, GIVEN THE RESOURCES AVAILABLE TO THEM.

A CLIENT'S BEHAVIOUR WILL always have a positive intention, even if the behaviour does not seem to be aligned with the intent the client has described to you. It's risky to criticise a client when it's the behaviour, not the person, that is to be critiqued. Discover what the intention was, and work with the client to help them find an action that's in line with their intention for the future.

For example, an individual may switch to a shake based liquid diet in order to lose weight. I hope that you'll agree with me that this is a terrible idea. We cannot critique the client, we can only critique the decision to only consume shakes, and even then, we need to be mindful that the client has made the decision based on the information found at the time.

I once took on a client whose previous personal trainer had told her that peanut butter before bed was good for weight loss. If you are told something by someone who's advice you've paid for, you're likely to believe it. Shit behaviour. Awesome client. She was only doing as she was told… Unfortunately for her, the resource available wasn't up to scratch. So, we critiqued that behaviour and we gave an action in line with the client's intention. I love peanut butter.

#84
YOU ARE NOT WALKING THE RED CARPET.

One of the diseases of our generation is to focus on how something seems – as opposed to how it is. Too many personal trainers are walking around like their album just went platinum, when the client's objectives should be their focus. My barber Andy once said to me, "Your haircut should look its best the minute it's been cut; people should leave the chair with their hair looking its best." I thought, "It's a shame people can't leave one session of personal training looking their best." Then I realised, they CAN leave their session 'feeling' their best. Your clients should leave their sessions feeling yes, fatigued, but more importantly, feeling accomplished and awesome. Make this the priority, not you gaining a little ego top-up so you can carry your invisible carpet home.

#85

STUDY MORE THAN EXERCISE AND NUTRITION.

Surprise your clients by being well versed in a variety of areas. Read, listen and study outside of fitness and nutrition. Look to learn other areas like sleep, stress, habitual patterns, emotional intelligence and hormonal profiles, to name a few. Having breadth of knowledge is never a bad thing and you never know what your clients are going to ask you.

#86

KEEP IT SIMPLE.

COMPLICATED PROGRAMS CAN be overwhelming for Olympic athletes – let alone beginners. Rather than showing off the latest periodisation, keep things simple for your client and avoid unnecessary difficulty and stress. It's very easy to get over excited by the latest nutrition protocol and foist it on an individual for whom it's just not required. More often than not, our clients are buying progress, not innovative exercises or ideologies.

#87

THE LAST CLIENT'S PROGRAM PRODUCED THE LAST CLIENT'S RESULTS.

Be wary of becoming lazy. When you're busy and have back- to-back sessions, there can be the temptation to repeat what you just did with the last client. Avoid this, for yourself as much as the client. Training people will become monotonous for you if you train them all the same. Yes, there are fundamental movement patterns that everyone can benefit from. Yes, if clients have similar goals, they may receive similar programs. However, even if a session or program was successful for one person, it can still be adapted, improved or made more specific for the next.

With the rise of online training, the amount of individualisation in programs has dropped. Individualisation is one of the key aspects that makes personal training *personal* training. This is not a copy-and-paste job.

#88
CARD-WORTHY.

WHEN YOUR CLIENTS sign up, take note of their birthday. Be sure to give them a card. You can set this up automatically on a few of the popular card selling websites, or even hand-write one yourself. I hate the 'extra mile' chat, but this is the extra mile. They're investing in you, so a card will mean more to them than that two quid still in your pocket.

#89

REWARD LONGEVITY AND GOAL SUCCESS.

Your clients are an advertisement for you. The longer they've been using your service, the longer they've been advertising for you. If they've stayed committed to you, they must have had some goal success, whether a small or big win. That testimonial advertises you. Reward this.

You are a service business, so reward loyalty and commitment. Coffee shops, health clubs and restaurants do this well. Back in the day, there was a Nando's loyalty card. When I went in knowing I was on a free whole chicken, I felt like a VIP. Find your equivalent.

#90

STICK 'EM UP!

One of the most common mistakes I've seen new personal trainers make is undervaluing their services. If you've made this mistake, don't be afraid to correct it and re-structure your pricing. Give your clients a notice period, so that they can adjust. Don't leave yourself undervalued.

If your books are full and you don't wish to work any more hours, put your prices up. Continue this process every time you've been full for 3 months. There's no promotion as a personal trainer, so give yourself a raise.

#91

GET SOCIAL PROOF.

Years ago, collecting written client testimonials would be good advice. Today, the effort that it takes us to get a video or photo testimonial is so little that written words don't stand for much.

We live in such a visually stimulated world that before and after photos and interviews between yourself and your client – provided they're comfortable to do so – are always going to be a winner. Whether this is proof of weight loss, strength gain or endurance, the proof has got to be there.

Imagine you're getting a tattoo or having some dental alterations. You would certainly want to see that the person conducting the procedure has done it before.

#92

KNOW THE SIZE OF YOUR POND.

So, YOU'VE BUILT your client base. This is a big moment in a personal trainer's career as you realise, "Shit, I'm making money doing this!" Grasp what's around you and don't adopt an ego. As Ryan Holiday explains in his book *The Ego is the Enemy*, "People can be assholes and win. Anyone can win. But not everyone is the best possible version of themselves."

You'll often see a large ego on a personal trainer who has little competition in their location. Sure, be confident in yourself, but not at the expense of another trainer. Chin up, sit down, stay humble.

#93

CANCELLATION POLICY.

A 24-HOUR CANCELLATION POLICY is the usual practice for most personal trainers. This is where the client would be charged the full amount for the session if cancelled within 24 hours.

Within your usual week you can expect 10% of your sessions to get cancelled. Factor this into your weekly finance. If you expect it, it won't affect you.

Yes, your time is valuable. Yes, there's no point in a policy unless it's enforced. Yes, you must treat all clients the same.

Whilst this is a policy you need to have, don't be so quick to enforce it. Have an unspoken three strikes policy. Take into account illness and family emergencies. Of course, if there are repeat offenders, charge them.

If you act too quick to enforce this kind of policy, you have set a very high standard for yourself. Just remember there may come a day when you need to cancel a session.

#94

YOUR NICHE CAN BE YOU.

It's fantastic to have a direct skill to pass on, like being a powerlifting coach, a body building prep coach or even a handstand coach. How cool has the fitness industry become recently that we have handstand coaches? Hey, don't be concerned if you don't have a niche.

If there is a population that isn't being addressed, don't be afraid to get in there and create something for them. I have a friend who did exactly that. He set up group training for people preparing for obstacle course races, a fantastic idea.

Now, you may be apprehensive that you don't have or don't want a niche and, if that's so, no drama. Often, if you're more of a general practitioner, your niche becomes you. In other words, your personality, the way you address and speak to people and your quirky ways of making the potentially complicated simple can be your niche.

Hard-nosed coaches, who say it the way it is, often have fans and anti-fans. Whereas trainers that are more cautious with their message will have fans, anti-fans and people without an opinion. Notice the trainers speaking their mind only have one demographic that won't purchase or follow their work, whilst cautious trainers have two demographics, anti-fans and people without an opinion, that won't follow their work.

Lesson: be shamelessly the most authentic version of yourself to build the most devoted following. You are already a niche; you just need to show people.

#95
THE FRIEND ZONE.

As a trainer you need to remember why your clients invested in you. Now, I'm not saying that you can't be friends with your clients. Just ensure your trainer obligations stay intact. Don't allow the fact that you've become friends let either of you slack off from the goals you've created. Try not to over share confidences with regard to yourself or the facility you work in. Clients don't need to know that the gym manager is sleeping with the lifeguard. Your client should still love the facility and need not know the naughtiness that surrounds the fitness environment.

Don't allow the paid session to blur into a chat about weekend plans for you both. Maintain the intensity promised and keep your coaching duties, your coaching duties.

#96

'BUT' AND 'AND' REFRAMING.

In our speech the word 'and' is used to join sentences together or introduce another comment, potentially to highlight the value of the words said previously. For example, "I want to lose 12lbs and this time I'm going to keep it off." Often, our clients will tell us what they want, and then follow it with a big nasty "but …". 'But' in our speech is used to introduce a comment which contrasts with what was previously said. For example, "I want to lose 12lbs, but last time I didn't manage to keep it off." Usually in goal setting conversations the 'but' is the client's perceived barrier to their goal, or just a glimpse of pessimism toward the process.

Whilst we can't control what a client says, we can control what we say. When we're in consultation, pacing and leading the client towards what they want, delete 'but' from your communication, as we don't want to negate what we've said previously. We can use 'and' instead.

It's important to note that 'but' isn't necessarily a bad word; we just need to use it in a way that promotes progress. When we have a 'but' in a sentence, we need to put the most positive part of the statement at the end. This gets clients thinking in a more resourceful manner.

You could respond to your client reframing what they've said: "So, you didn't manage to keep it off last time, but you do want to lose 12lbs."

So, to keep our consultations goal-driven rather than excuse-driven, we can lead by using the word 'and', and reframe by having the action or positive part of a statement after the word 'but', when 'but' is being used.

#97

YOU MAY FALL OUT OF LOVE WITH YOUR TRAINING.

We give the gym the power to destroy us, trusting that it won't. This is exactly how writer Emily Lockhart describes Love: "... giving someone the power to destroy you but trusting them not to." We mustn't come into personal training with the preconceived notion being a personal training will make us immune to falling out of love with training.

When you've been working an 8-hour day, asking your body to train in the same room afterwards can be an internal battle. You have options, you can white knuckle it – no pain, no gain. You can schedule your own session before or amongst your clients in your diary, putting your oxygen mask on first, so to speak. You can look to get your own coach, learn some new skills, put part of the responsibility in someone else's hands. No shame. I'm sure Ronald McDonald's gone to Burger King when he was sick of big Macs.

These suggestions may not be the solution. Sometimes, it's just not happening. I've been there myself, many times in truth, feeling fraudulent as I action more reps, sets, minutes and effort. If and when you do start to fall out of love with your own training, as cliché as it sounds, you're not the first and you won't be the last. AND it's something that's only going to make you a stronger coach. I will add that 'often' when you don't want to, is perhaps when you need to the most.

#98

THE PRINCIPLES BUILD THE PLAN.

TEACH THE FUNDAMENTAL principles of fitness and nutrition to your clients as opposed to delivering just plans. A principle is a foundational truth that controls how something works. For example, progressive overload and energy balance are underpinning principles which will uphold successful training and 'diet' plans. There's no need not to let the client know why they're doing what they're doing.

#99

INCLUDE PLAY IN YOUR SESSIONS.

Adherence is the most important aspect of training. That is… actually turning up. Sometimes training is taken very seriously – rightly so, since it is our client's health we're dealing with after all. But at other times we do need to cut loose and have a giggle. Add some fun in and people are more likely to keep coming. At the end of a circuits class, group personal training session or couples training session add a bit of play in. There are loads of great examples on the internet – noughts and crosses, relays and ball and spoon races being my personal favourite.

#100

DON'T DISCUSS YOUR PRICES ON THE GYM FLOOR.

UNLESS YOUR PRICES are standardised in your workplace, don't discuss them on the gym floor. What your clients are paying you is private between you and them. Leave the gym floor for training.

#101

PERSEVERANCE AND PREPARING FOR NO END.

I SEE SO MANY good personal trainers leave the industry because they struggled to get clients. The biggest problem here is allowing the end of their fitness career to be an option. If being a personal trainer is really what you want, keep using trial and error until you work it all out. Don't let not getting what you want become an option. In a lot of cases, this career is harder than you think and is going to take more work and time than you imagined. However, I believe you'll get more reward than you believed possible.

Henry Ford said, "Whether you think you can or you think you can't, you're right." So, we need to focus our minds on what we want. My personal belief is that the personal trainers who struggle to carve their path long term have let the shitty committee in their head take over their thought process. Rather than thinking about what they want, they're thinking of why they can't, or measuring themselves against other people has led them to conclude that they can't. Perseverance is often the only way. Like training weights, we have the option of using advanced techniques, when we know it's the progressive overload that will get us the strength, endurance or the physique we desire.

Give yourself permission to fail as from now. Failure is just feedback. Consider failure your first attempt at learning. Don't give yourself the option to quit. As soon as you put the quitting card in the slot, it will become all too easy to play it. So, what are you going to do? Fixate on what you want, with a mindset that's happy to endure trial and error, and a passion that outweighs the comforts that may lie elsewhere. Do this and, as you did as a toddler, crawls will become walks, walks will become runs, runs will become jumps and jumps will become options. Once you've completed perseverance, you inherit tenacity. Tenacity is 'the quality or fact of being able to grip something firmly'. So, persevere and you will get a grip on being the coach you envisaged.

CLOSING STATEMENT

PHWOAR… THAT DIDN'T touch the sides did it?! Lolz, I hope you enjoyed my book. As I expressed at the beginning, it may not have all been for you, but I'm sure that there's something for you to take on board and add to yourself as a coach.

A message I really want to fixate on is focusing on what you want, as nothing can be gained from focusing on anything else.

Keep learning, keep reading and keep succeeding.

I'm contactable in the following places:

Instagram: @thepttrainer

Email: Oli.smallwood@thepttrainer.co.uk

I'd love to hear your thoughts.

Again, thank you for reading.

Printed in Great Britain
by Amazon

83867679R00078